A BEGINNER'S GUIDE TO COOKING FOR CANCER PATIENTS.

Nourishing Your Body And Soul : The Power Of Food in The Fight Against Cancer.

JENNIFER M.LUX

COPYRIGHT PAGE.

All rights reserved. No part of the publication may be reproduced, distributed or transmitted, including by photocopying, recording or by any other means electronic or mechanical, without the prior written permission by copyright law.

Copyright by JENNIFER M.LUX 2023.

TABLE OF CONTENTS.

CHAPTER ONE.
INTRODUCTION.
_What is cancer ?

CHAPTER TWO.
OVERVIEW OF A BEGINNER'S GUIDE TO COOKING FOR CANCER PATIENTS.
_What is A Beginner' s GuIde To Cooking For Cancer Patients ?
_Why use a Beginner's Guide To Cooking For Cancer Patients Book. ?
_What kinds of recipes are there in A Beginner's Guide To Cooking For Cancer Patients Book ?

CHAPTER THREE.
UNDERSTANDING THE BASICS OF HEALTHY EATING FOR CANCER PATIENTS.
_Tips for eating a healthy diet during cancer treatment.
_Tips for meal planning grocery shopping for cancer patients.
_Importance of a balanced diet for cancer patients.
_ The secrets of tomatoes to cancer patients.
_Homemade butter and nuts .

CHAPTER FOUR.
CANCER MEAL PLAN .

CHAPTER FIVE.

FOODS TO EAT AND FOODS TO AVOID DURING CANCER TREATMENT.
_Foods to eat during cancer treatment.
_Foods to avoid during cancer treatment.

CHAPTER SIX.
CANCER RECIPES.
_Breakfast.
_Lunch
_Dinner.
_Smoothie.
_7 meal plan days.
_Snacks
_Other simple recipes for cancer patients.

CHAPTER SEVEN.
CONCLUSION.

CHAPTER ONE.
INTRODUCTION.

Cancer is a disease that affects millions of people worldwide. It can be a challenging and overwhelming experience for both patients and their loved ones.

Cancer is a disease characterized by the uncontrolled growth and spread of abnormal cells throughout the body. These cells can be found with the tumor, invade surrounding tissues, and spread to other parts of the body through the bloodstream and lymphatic system, there are many different types of cancer, each with its own symptoms, treatment outcomes.

One of the most important aspects of cancer treatment is maintaining a healthy diet. Eating well can help boost your immune system, reduce side effects of treatment, and improve your overall quality of life. However, it can be difficult to know what to eat and how to prepare healthy meals, especially if you're new to cooking or have dietary restrictions.

That's where A Beginners Guide To Cooking For Cancer Patients comes in. This cookbook is designed to provide you with delicious and nutritious recipes that are easy to prepare and tailored to the needs of cancer patients and survivors. Whether you're looking for quick and easy meals or more elaborate dishes, this cookbook has something for everyone.

The recipes in this cookbook are based on the latest research on cancer and nutrition. We've included ingredients that are known to have cancer-fighting properties, such as fruits, vegetables, whole grains, and lean proteins. We've also taken into account common side effects of cancer treatment, such as nausea, fatigue, and loss of appetite, and have included recipes that are gentle on the stomach and easy to digest.

Cancer is a disease that affects millions of people around the world. It can be a difficult and confusing experience for patients and their loved ones. One of the challenges that cancer patients face is maintaining a healthy diet during treatment. Eating well can help manage symptoms, improve energy levels, and support the body's immune system. This cookbook is designed for beginners looking for simple, nutritious recipes that can help support their health during cancer treatment. The recipes in this cookbook are easy to prepare, delicious, and packed with nutrients that can help boost your immune system and promote healing. In this cookbook, you will find many recipes designed to meet the unique needs of cancer patients. From smoothies and soups to appetizers and desserts, there is something for everyone. Each recipe includes an ingredient list, step-by-step instructions, and nutritional information. We understand cancer treatment can be overwhelming, which is why we've included tips and tricks for meal planning, shopping, and cooking. We hope this cookbook makes mealtime a little easier and more enjoyable for cancer patients and their loved ones.

Remember, healthy eating is only one part of an overall cancer treatment plan.

If you or a loved one has been diagnosed with cancer, it can be difficult to know what to eat. A healthy diet is important for everyone, but it is especially important for people undergoing cancer treatment. Eating well can help manage side effects, increase energy levels, and support overall health.

A Beginner's Guide To Cooking For Cancer Patients is designed to provide you with delicious, nutritious recipes that are easy to prepare and packed with cancer-fighting nutrients. From lunch to dinner, snacks to desserts, you'll find a variety of recipes that will satisfy your taste buds and support your health.

Here are some tips to keep in mind when using this cookbook:

Firstly, Focus on whole foods:

And choose foods that are minimally processed and nutrient-dense. This includes fruits, vegetables, whole grains, lean protein, and healthy fats. 2. Incorporate Diversity: Eating a variety of foods ensures that you get many of the nutrients your body needs. Try new recipes and experiment with different ingredients.

3. Stay hydrated: It is important to drink plenty of water and other fluids to stay hydrated and support the body's natural detoxification process.

4. Listen to Your Body: The Nutritional needs of everyone.

Once, Sarah was diagnosed with cancer. She is devastated and scared, but she knows she has to fight with everything she has. she started to learn and learn everything.

Maybe about cancer and its treatments. One day, Sarah came across this book, A Beginners Guide To Cooking For Cancer Patients .

She read it from start to finish and realized she ate it wrong. She decided to completely change her diet. Sarah started cooking all of her meals from scratch, using fresh ingredients. Avoid processed foods, sugar and unhealthy fats. Instead, eat plenty of fruits, vegetables, whole grains, and lean protein. It was tough at first. Sarah lacks familiar foods and craves sweets. But soon, she discovered new recipes and flavors that she loved. She also noticed that her energy levels improved and she felt better in general. After a few months of eating this way, Sarah went back to the doctor for a check-up. To her surprise, the doctor told her that her cancer had been cured. The tumor shrank and blood tests showed that her body was fighting the disease. Sarah is very happy. She knows her diet plays a huge role in her recovery. She continued to eat healthy, nutritious foods and even started sharing her recipes with other cancer patients. In the end, Sarah not only defeated cancer, but also discovered a new passion for cooking and living healthy. She knew she had made a difference in her life and the lives of others.

With this book in hand, you can boost your immune system.

WHAT IS A CANCER ?

Cancer is not an exclusive disease, but a group of diseases. It directly affects the growth of abnormal cells. They grow in large numbers and attack our immune system. Our bodies are living and dead cells. It is full of new cells. This cycle continues throughout life, but in cancer these cells do not die and continue to grow in large numbers. It is not needed by the body, but it is always present in it. It is important to get a timely diagnosis to prevent invasion. There are more than 100 different types of cancer known to man. It can occur in both men and women. Some are sexual because one organ is not present in the other. Two common examples are breast cancer in women and prostate cancer in men. There is no specific cause for cancer. It occurs when there are changes in the DNA of cells. This DNA is found in a large number of genes that require cells to perform certain functions. But when there is confusion, the cell has the potential to become cancerous. Not only does it allow these cells to grow rapidly, but it also cannot stop their uncontrolled growth. There are two main causes of genetic mutations:

Congenital mutations.

These mutations are present in the body from birth. You were born with them and you can inherit from your parents. But only a small percentage of cancers cause it.

Mutations formed after birth.
These are large in number and shape after birth. This may be due to lifestyle choices or side effects of certain diseases. The most dangerous thing about cancer is that there is no identifiable cause. There are many risk factors associated with this disease, but staying away from all of them can also cause cancer.

Some common risk factors are as follows:
• Age

Many types of cancer take a long time for symptoms to appear and for them to appear. They can stay in the body for a while, but symptoms only appear when they are in an advanced stage.
1.Many lifestyles are risk factors. These include smoking and drinking alcohol regularly.
2.Excessive exposure to the skin is a major cause of skin cancer. It causes burns and blisters on the body.
3. A small percentage of cancers are also inherited from family members. The risk increases if one or more members of the system are affected.
4.Obesity causes many weight problems directly related to the disease. Fat cells in the

body manage the processes that regulate the growth of cancer cells.

5. The environment also has some problems. Even if you don't smoke, breathing in secondhand smoke can be harmful.

6. Regular cancer screening is recommended if any of the above risk factors are suspected to be relevant to you.

Common treatments are
Equal:
This treatment uses medicines to destroy the growth of cancer cells. In this treatment, one drug or a combination of drugs is used. But because it kills cells so quickly, it can also damage some nearby cells. It may be given before or after surgery, or as the only way.

Radiotherapy
It destroys infected cells through the use of high-energy X-rays and other radiation methods. More than half of people with cancer receive radiation therapy at one time or another.

Surgery
Surgery is an operation to remove the tumor. The goals of surgery vary. It is not only used to treat diseases but also to diagnose diseases in the body. Staging is a type of surgery that is done to see how far the cancer has spread .

CHAPTER TWO.
OVERVIEW OF A BEGINNER'S GUIDE TO COOKING FOR CANCER PATIENTS.

A Beginner's Guide To Cooking For Cancer Patients is a cookbook aimed at those newly diagnosed with cancer who may be struggling to eat healthy. This cookbook contains easy_to_make recipes designed to help people maintain energy levels and stay healthy during cancer treatment. A cancer diagnosis can leave patients feeling overwhelmed and helpless. However, it is important to remember that there are many ways to take control of your health during cancer treatment. One of these ways is to eat a healthy diet. A beginners cancer cookbook can give patients the tools they need to create healthy, nutritious meals that support their bodies during treatment.

What is A Beginner's Guide To Cooking For Cancer Patients ?

A Beginner's Guide To Cooking For Cancer Patients is a collection of recipes that are specifically designed to help people with cancer maintain a healthy diet. The recipes in these cookbooks are often created with the guidance of nutrition experts and oncologists to ensure that they are both delicious and nutritious.

A Beginner's Guide To Cooking For Cancer Patients can help patients manage side effects of cancer treatment, such as fatigue, nausea, and loss of appetite, and they can also provide a sense of control and comfort in their lives.

Why Use A Beginner's Guide To Cooking For Cancer Patients ?

Cancer treatment can be physically and mentally stressful. Patients often experience a variety of side effects that can make it difficult to eat and enjoy food. A Beginner's Guide To Cooking For Cancer Patients can provide patients with recipes that are easy to prepare, healthy, and delicious. These prescriptions can help patients maintain their strength and energy levels during cancer treatment, and can also help them feel more in control of their health.

What Kinds Of Recipes Are There in A Beginner's Guide To Cooking For Cancer Patients ?

A Beginner's Guide To Cooking For Cancer Patients often includes many recipes tailored to the needs of cancer patients. These recipes may include:

_Lightweight and Easy-to-digest meals .

protein recipes to help maintain muscle mass

- Nutrient-rich foods that support the immune system

A formula that combines cancer_fighting foods, such as vegetables and berries,low sugar and low fat recipes help control blood sugar.

Moisturizing Formula to combat dryness , light recipes to help patients maintain energy level throughout the day.

Recipes are easy to prepare and can be made in large batches for convenience.

Here are some tips for creating A Beginner's Guide To Cooking For Cancer Patients.

1:Focus on nutritious foods: Nutritious foods are foods rich in vitamins, minerals and other nutrients that are important for Maintaining good health.A Beginners Guide To Cooking For Cancer Patients recommends fruits, vegetables, whole grain and lean protein.

2: Accommodates a variety of tastes: People undergoing cancer treatment may notice changes in taste, Therefore,it is important to include different flavors in your recipes.This makes eating more enjoyable and also stimulates appetite.

3:Consider Diet: Many people undergoing cancer treatment may be on a diet due to treatment or other health conditions. A Beginner's Guide To Cooking For Cancer Patients should contain recipes suitable for different diets such as low fat,low sugar,or gluten free etc.

4:Provide helpful recipe tips: A Beginner's Guide To Cooking For Cancer Patients should also include helpful tips and resources for Maintaining a healthy diet during cancer treatment.This include information about portion sizes,meal plans, and other strategies for maintaining a good diet.

Overall, A Beginner's Guide To Cooking For Cancer Patients can be a valuable resource for anyone undergoing cancer treatment. The cancer cookbook helps people stay healthy and happy during the challenging time by focusing on nutritious foods with a variety of flavors while addressing dietary restrictions.

CHAPTER THREE.
UNDERSTANDING THE BASICS OF HEALTHY EATING FOR CANCER PATIENTS.

Understanding the basics of healthy eating for cancer patients involves a holistic approach that takes into account the unique nutritional needs of people undergoing cancer treatment. This includes emphasizing a well-balanced diet rich in nutrients, vitamins, and minerals, and limiting consumption of processed foods, added sugars, and unhealthy fats. A healthy diet for cancer patients should include a variety of fruits, vegetables, whole grains, lean proteins, and healthy fats. It is also important to stay hydrated by drinking plenty of water and other fluids. In addition to a balanced diet, cancer patients can also benefit from working with a registered dietitian who can provide personalized nutrition advice and support. This may include creating a meal plan that takes into account dietary restrictions or side effects of cancer treatment, as well as advice on how to manage symptoms such as nausea, vomiting, and boredom. Overall, understanding the basics of healthy eating for cancer patients involves a holistic approach that prioritizes providing the body with nutrient-dense foods, taking into account the patient's needs and the unique needs and challenges of cancer treatment.

Understanding the fundamentals of healthy eating for cancer patients requires a comprehensive approach that considers the particular nutritional requirements of individuals. This entails putting an emphasis on eating a diet that is well-balanced, full of nutrients, vitamins, and minerals, and avoiding processed foods, added sweets, and bad fats.

Cancer patients should consume a variety of fruits, vegetables, whole grains, lean proteins, and healthy fats as part of a nutritious diet. Drinking plenty of water and other drinks will help you stay hydrated. Cancer patients can gain from working with a licensed dietitian who can offer individualized nutrition guidance and assistance in addition to eating a balanced diet. This can entail making a meal plan that considers dietary limitations or adverse effects.

Eating healthy and balanced is important for cancer patients. A healthy diet can help manage symptoms, improve energy levels, and support the body's immune system. Include a variety of fruits and vegetables in your diet to ensure you're getting a variety of nutrients.

Choose lean protein sources such as chicken, fish and legumes.Limit saturated and trans fats foods such as fried foods, fatty meats and baked goods.

Choose whole grains for bread, pasta, and rice to increase your fiber intake.

Limit your intake of sugary drinks such as sodas and juices.

Read food labels carefully to understand the ingredients and nutritional value of the foods you eat.

Here are some basics of healthy eating for cancer patients:

1. Eat a variety of foods: Eating a variety of foods can help ensure that you are getting all the nutrients your body needs. Include fruits,

vegetables, whole grains, lean proteins, and healthy fats in your diet.

2.Choose nutrient-dense foods: Nutrient-dense foods are foods that are high in nutrients but low in calories. Examples include leafy greens, berries, nuts, and seeds.

3. Reduced Processed foods: Foods processed such as,,high proportion of sugar,sait and unhealthy fats,Limit intake of processed foods and choose whole, unprocessed foods whenever possible.

4. Stay hydrated: Drinking enough water is important for everyone, but it is especially important for cancer patients. Aim to drink at least 8-10 glasses of water per day.

5. Consider supplements: Some cancer treatments can affect the body's ability to absorb nutrients. Talk to your doctor or a registered dietitian about whether you should know or learn about cancer.

Tips For Eating A Healthy Diet During Cancer Treatment.

A healthy diet is important for everyone but it is especially important for cancer patients.cancer treatment can have a number of side effects that make it difficult to eat healthy.These side effects may include:
Anorexia ,Vomiting and diarrhea,
Diarrhea holding mouth ulcers,
Changes in the sense of taste exhausted.These side effects can make it difficult to absorb nutrients needed to stay healthy and fight cancer. A healthy diet can help you maintain a healthy weight,
Build strength,reduce the risk of infection, Improve your mood dealing
with the side effects of treatment.
There is no single diet for cancer. The best diet for you will depend on your individual needs and preferences. However, there are some general guidelines that can help you create a healthy diet.

1:Eat plenty of fruits and vegetables. Fruits and vegetables are full of vitamins, minerals, and antioxidants that can help you fight cancer.
2:Choose lean protein sources. Lean protein sources, such as fish, chicken, and beans, can help you build strength and maintain muscle mass.
3:Limit processed foods. Processed foods are often high in unhealthy fats, sugars and salts. These

foods can contribute to weight gain, inflammation, and other health problems.

4:Drink a lot of water: Fluids are important for staying hydrated and removing toxins from your body.

If you are having trouble eating a healthy diet, talk to your doctor or a registered dietitian. They can help you create a plan that meets your individual needs.

Here are some additional tips for eating a healthy diet during cancer treatment:

Eat several small, frequent meals throughout the day. This can help you avoid feeling too full or too hungry.

Choose foods that are easy to digest. These foods include soft cooked vegetables, lean meats, and whole grains.

Avoid foods that are spicy, fatty, or acidic foods. These foods can irritate your stomach and make it difficult for you to eat them.

Drink a lot of water: Fluids help keep your body hydrated and can help to flush toxins from your system.

Talk to your doctor or a registered dietitian about any specific dietary concerns you may have.

Healthy eating can be a challenge during cancer treatment, but it is important to make the effort . Eating healthy can help you stay healthy and fight cancer.

Tips For Meal Planning Grocery Shopping For Cancer Patients.

Consult with a registered dietitian or nutritionist: They can help develop a balanced and nutritious meal plan that is suitable for the specific cancer patient's needs.

It is always best to consult a registered dietitian who specializes in oncology nutrition for specialized advice, as they can provide personalized recommendations tailored to the patient's specific needs.

2. **Plan for Nutrient-rich Foods:** Opt for nutrient-dense meals including fruits, vegetables, whole grains, lean proteins, and healthy fats, which can help boost the immune system and also help prevent cancer from recurring.

Focus on whole foods, Plan meals that center around fresh fruits, vegetables, whole grains, lean proteins, and healthy fats. Avoid processed and packaged foods, as they often contain high levels of salt, sugar, and unhealthy fats.

3. **Incorporate Anti-inflammatory Foods:**
Foods high in antioxidants and anti-inflammatory properties such as berries, leafy greens, turmeric, ginger, and oily fish like salmon can help reduce inflammation and support healing, include plenty of antioxidants:

Antioxidants can help protect cells from damage caused by cancer and its treatment. Foods that are high in antioxidants include berries, dark leafy greens, nuts, and seeds.

4. Keep it Simple:
Focus on simple, quick, and easy-to-digest meals to avoid any digestive issues that can occur during cancer treatment.

5. Consider Supplements:
Discuss with the patient's healthcare team if any vitamin or mineral supplements may be helpful.

6. Prioritize Food Safety:
Patients with cancer may have a weakened immune system, making them more susceptible to foodborne illness. Proper food handling and storage, as well as avoiding potentially contaminated foods, can help reduce the risk of infections.

7. Shop mindfully: When grocery shopping, read labels carefully and choose foods that are low in sugar, salt, and unhealthy fats. Try to buy fresh, organic produce when possible.
Opt for fresh, unprocessed foods and avoid pre-packaged and processed foods, which can be high in sodium, sugar, and unhealthy fats.

8. Plan Ahead:

Plan meals for the week ahead of time and make a list of the required ingredients. This saves time, money, and helps prevent impulse buying.

It's helpful to plan meals ahead of time and make a grocery list to ensure that all necessary ingredients are on hand. This can also save time and reduce stress during the week.

9. Avoid Food Wastage:
Plan meals based on the patient's appetite and preferences to avoid food wastage. Use leftovers for future meals or freeze them for later use.

10. Consider Home Delivery:
To avoid public places during treatment, consider using a grocery delivery service to ensure that the patient has access to fresh and healthy foods.

11. Be mindful of food safety: Cancer patients are often more susceptible to infections, so it's crucial to take extra precautions when handling food. Wash fresh produce thoroughly, cook meats thoroughly, and avoid consuming raw or undercooked foods.

12. Consider special dietary needs: Cancer patients may have specific dietary needs, such as avoiding certain foods or increasing their

intake of particular nutrients. Consult with a healthcare provider or dietitian to determine the patient's particular needs.

Importance of a balanced diet for cancer patients.

Although there are many different types of cancer, one thing is consistent across all forms of the disease and that is the importance of a well-balanced diet for cancer patients. A well-balanced diet can help support the body's immune system, reduce inflammation, and provide nutrients needed to help fight cancer and manage the side effects of cancer treatment.

A well-balanced cancer diet should include a variety of foods from all the major food groups, including fruits, vegetables, whole grains, lean proteins, and healthy fats. These foods provide the body with the nutrients it needs to function properly, including vitamins, minerals, antioxidants, and fiber.

Fruits and vegetables are especially important for cancer patients, as they are rich in antioxidants and other compounds that can help reduce inflammation and support the immune system. Some studies also suggest that certain fruits and vegetables may have cancer-fighting properties, making them an important part of a cancer-fighting diet.

Whole grains are another important component of a balanced diet for cancer patients. These foods are high in fiber, which may help promote healthy digestion and reduce the risk of certain types of cancer, such as colon cancer. Whole grains also provide the body with important vitamins.

A balanced diet is essential for everyone, but it is even more important for cancer patients. It's no secret that cancer treatment can take a toll on the body, both physically and mentally. A well-balanced diet can help cancer patients maintain their strength and energy to deal with the side effects of cancer treatment. One of the most important reasons why cancer patients should eat a balanced diet is to support the body's immune system. A healthy, balanced diet that provides essential nutrients can help the body fight cancer cells and boost the immune system. A diet low in nutrients can make the body more susceptible to infection, making it harder to fight cancer cells.

Another reason why a well-balanced diet is essential for cancer patients is maintaining a healthy weight. Some cancer patients may experience weight loss or gain during treatment, which may affect their general health and wellness. A well-balanced diet can help cancer patients maintain their weight and prevent further weight loss, which can lead to weakness and fatigue. Cancer patients can also benefit from a balanced diet by reducing inflammation in the body. Inflammation can contribute to the growth of cancer cells, and a diet high in processed foods, sugar, and unhealthy fats can increase inflammation. On the other hand, a diet rich in fruits, vegetables, whole grains, and lean protein can reduce inflammation and promote healing.

Ultimately, a well-balanced diet can improve the quality of life for cancer patients. A nutrient-dense diet can help cancer patients feel more energetic, improve mental clarity, and lower their risk of other chronic diseases. By eating a well-balanced diet, cancer patients can take control of their health and improve their overall health. In short, a well-balanced diet is essential for cancer patients to maintain strength, energy, and general health during cancer treatment. A nutrient-dense diet can strengthen the immune system, maintain a healthy weight, reduce inflammation, and improve the quality of life for cancer patients. By working with a registered dietitian, people with cancer can create a personalized nutrition plan that meets their individual needs and supports their overall health and well-being.

THE SECRETS OF TOMATOES TO CANCER PATIENTS.

Here are good secrets of tomatoes to cancer patients:

Tomatoes are a good source of lycopene, an antioxidant that has been shown to protect against cancer. Lycopene is a carotenoid, which is a type of pigment that gives tomatoes their red color. It is also found in other fruits and vegetables, such as watermelon, pink grapefruit, and apricots.

Studies have shown that people who eat a lot of tomatoes have a lower risk of developing certain types of cancer, such as prostate cancer, lung cancer, and stomach cancer. In one study, men who ate the most tomatoes had a 35% lower risk of developing prostate cancer than men who ate the least tomatoes.

The lycopene in tomatoes can help to protect cells from damage by free radicals. Free radicals are unstable molecules that can damage cells and lead to cancer. Lycopene can help to neutralize free radicals and prevent them from damaging cells.

Tomatoes also contain other nutrients that may help to fight cancer, such as vitamin C, vitamin E, and potassium. Vitamin C is an antioxidant that can help to protect cells from damage. Vitamin E is also an antioxidant, and it can help to boost the immune system. Potassium is a mineral that can help to regulate blood pressure, which is a risk factor for cancer.

In addition to their anti-cancer benefits, tomatoes are also a good source of fiber, vitamins, and minerals. Fiber can help to keep you feeling full and can help to regulate digestion. Vitamins and minerals are essential for good health, and they can help to boost the immune system.

If you are a cancer patient, it is important to eat a healthy diet that includes plenty of fruits, vegetables, and whole grains. Tomatoes are a good choice for cancer patients because they are a good source of lycopene and other nutrients that may help to fight cancer.

You can eat tomatoes in a variety of ways. You can eat them raw, cooked, or juiced. You can also add them to salads, soups, stews, and sauces.

If you are taking medication, be sure to talk to your doctor before adding tomatoes to your diet. Some medications can interact with lycopene, so it is important to be safe.

Here are some additional tips for cancer patients who want to get the most benefits from tomatoes:

Choose tomatoes that are red, ripe, and firm.
Avoid canned tomatoes that are high in sodium.
Cook tomatoes with a small amount of olive oil or water to help your body absorb the lycopene.
Eat tomatoes with other foods that are high in vitamin C, such as citrus fruits or broccoli.
Drink tomato juice or eat tomato soup on a regular basis.

By following these tips, you can help to boost your intake of lycopene and other nutrients that may help to fight cancer.

HOMEMADE BUTTER AND NUTS.

2.Nuts and nut butters are not only delicious, but also a great source of healthy fats, protein, and other essential nutrients. For cancer patients, homemade nut butters and nuts can be a great way to incorporate healthy fats and protein into their diet. Here are some easy homemade nut butter and nut butter recipes that cancer patients may love:

1.Almond Butter.

Ingredients
- 2 cups of raw almonds
1-2 teaspoons sea salt (optional)
1-2 tablespoons of coconut oil (optional)

Instructions

Firstly, Preheat the oven to 350oC.
2.Spread the almonds on a baking sheet and bake for 10-12 minutes or until lightly browned and fragrant.
3. Let the almonds cool for a few minutes, then transfer them to a food processor.
4.Blend the almonds for 5-10 minutes or until the mixture is smooth and creamy.
5.Add the salt and coconut oil (if using) and mix again until well combined.
6.Store the almond butter in an airtight container in the refrigerator for up to 2 weeks.

2. Cashew Butter.

Ingredients
- 2 cups of raw cashews
1-2 teaspoons sea salt (optional)
1-2 tablespoons of coconut oil (optional)

Instructions
1. Preheat the oven to 350oC.
2. Spread the cashews on the baking tray and bake for 10-12 minutes or until light brown and fragrant.
3. Let the cashews cool for a few minutes and then place them in a food processor.
4. Grind the cashews for 5-10 minutes or until the mixture becomes smooth and creamy.
5. Add salt and coconut oil (if using) and mix again until combined.
6. Store the cashew butter in an airtight container in the refrigerator for up to 2 weeks.

3. Sunflower Seed Butter.

Ingredients
2 cups of raw sunflower seeds
1-2 teaspoons sea salt (optional)
1-2 tablespoons of coconut oil (optional)

Instructions
Firstly, Preheat the oven to 350oC.
2. Spread the sunflower seeds on a baking sheet and bake for 10-12 minutes or until lightly browned and fragrant.

3. Let the sunflower seeds cool for a few minutes, then transfer them to a food processor.
4. Grind the sunflower seeds for 5-10 minutes or until the mixture is smooth and creamy.
5. Add the salt and coconut oil (if using) and mix again until well combined.
6. Store sunflower seed butter in an airtight container in the refrigerator for up to 2 weeks.

Homemade nut butters and nuts are not only delicious, but they are also a great source of healthy fats and protein, which may benefit cancer patients. They can be used as a spread on toast, added to smoothies, or used as a dipping sauce for fruits and vegetables. Always consult a registered dietitian before making any changes to your diet.

CHAPTER FOUR.
CANCER MEAL PLAN.

A cancer meal plan is a diet plan designed to meet the nutritional needs of people undergoing cancer treatment. This often includes incorporating nutrient-dense foods that can help boost your immune system, manage treatment side effects, and maintain a healthy weight. Your cancer meal plan may also include avoiding certain foods that can interfere with treatment or worsen side effects. The goal of a cancer meal plan is to provide the body with the nutrients it needs to support general health and well-being throughout the cancer treatment journey.

It is important to note that the nutritional needs of cancer patients vary according to the type of cancer, its stage, and the treatment plan. Therefore, it is highly recommended that you consult a medical professional before following any particular diet plan.

CHAPTER FIVE.
FOODS TO EAT AND AVOID DURING CANCER TREATMENT.

Foods To Eat During Cancer Treatment.

1. Fruits and vegetables:

These are rich in vitamins, minerals, and antioxidants that help support the immune system and fight cancer cells.**Fresh fruits and vegetables are full of essential vitamins, minerals and antioxidants that may help boost the immune system and fight cancer. Some of the best choices include leafy greens, berries, citrus fruits, squash, and cruciferous vegetables like broccoli and cauliflower.**

2. Whole grains:

These provide fiber and nutrients that help keep the body healthy and prevent inflammation.

Replace refined grains with whole grains such as brown rice, quinoa, and whole grain breads, pastas, and cereals. Whole grains are high in fiber and can help regulate digestion and maintain a healthy weight.

3. Lean protein:

This includes chicken, fish, eggs, and legumes that provide essential amino acids for building and repairing tissues.

Choose lean protein sources such as fish, chicken, beans and lentils because they are low in fat and provide essential nutrients that can aid in the recovery process

4. Healthy fats:
These include avocados, nuts, seeds, and olive oil that provide omega-3 fatty acids and other nutrients that support brain health and reduce inflammation. Certain types of fats, such as omega-3 fatty acids, found in fish, flaxseeds, and nuts, can help reduce inflammation and promote heart health.

5. Water:
Staying hydrated is important for overall health and helps flush out toxins from the body.

6. Cruciferous vegetables:
Vegetables such as broccoli, cauliflower, and kale contain compounds that may help prevent cancer and reduce inflammation.

7. Berries:
Berries like blueberries, strawberries, and raspberries are rich in antioxidants that may help protect cells from cancer damage.

8. Green Tea:
It contains compounds that have been shown to reduce the risk of cancer and improve overall health.

9. Mushrooms:
Some types of mushrooms such as shiitake and maitake contain compounds that may help boost the immune system and fight cancer cells.

10. Herbs and spices:
Adding herbs and spices like turmeric, ginger and garlic to your meals can provide anti-inflammatory and antioxidant benefits.

Foods To Avoid During Cancer Treatment.
1.Processed and packaged foods: They often contain preservatives, additives and chemicals that can increase the risk of cancer.

2.High-fat dairy products:
These products can contribute to inflammation in the body and increase the risk of certain types of cancer.

3.Refined carbohydrates:
Foods such as white bread, pasta, and rice can cause blood sugar to spike and promote inflammation in the body.

4.Artificial sweeteners:
They can upset the balance of healthy gut bacteria and increase your risk of certain types of cancer.

5. Processed meats:
These contain chemicals that can increase the risk of cancer.Processed **foods like packaged snacks, fast foods, and sugary drinks are often high in unhealthy fats, sugars, and salts, which can**

contribute to inflammation and increase your risk of cancer.

6. Sugary drinks and snacks:
These can cause inflammation in the body and increase the risk of obesity, which is a risk factor for many types of cancer.

7. Alcohol:
This can damage cells and increase the risk of several types of cancer. **Drinking alcohol can increase your risk of certain types of cancer, including breast cancer and liver cancer. If you drink alcohol, drink in moderation and talk to your doctor about the risks.**

8. Fried and grilled foods:
These can produce harmful chemicals when cooked at high temperatures.

9. Foods high in saturated and trans fats:
These can increase inflammation in the body and contribute to the development of cancer.
Saturated **fats and trans fats found in fried foods, baked goods and some margarines can increase inflammation and contribute to heart disease and cancer. Reduce your intake of these fats and choose healthy alternatives.**
It is important for cancer patients to consult with their healthcare providers and dietitian to develop an individualized nutrition plan.

10.Red and processed meat:
Red meat, especially when it is processed, is associated with an increased risk of colon cancer. Limit your intake of beef, pork and lamb, and choose lean cuts of meat. Eating a lot of red meat is linked to an increased risk of colorectal cancer.

CHAPTER SIX.
CANCER RECIPES.

BREAKFAST.
1. Oatmeal with chopped nuts and berries.
2. Greek yogurt with honey and granola.
3. Scrambled eggs with spinach and whole grains toast.
4. Smoothie Bowl With Mixed Berries And Chia Seeds.
5. Avocado Toast With Smoked Salmon.
6. Quinoa breakfast bowl with fruit and nuts.
7. Whole grain waffles with peanut butter and banana.
8. Breakfast Burrito with scrambled eggs and black beans.
9. Cottage cheese with fruit and honey.
10. Veggie omelet with whole grain toast.

_Oatmeal With Chopped Nuts And Berries.

Ingredients
- 1 cup of hard oats
- 2 cups of almond milk
1/4 cup chopped nuts (such as almonds or walnuts)
1/2 cup fresh berries (such as blueberries or strawberries)

instructions
1. In a medium saucepan, bring the almond milk to a boil.

2. Add the rolled oats, mix well and reduce heat.
3. Simmer for 20 minutes, stirring occasionally, until the oats are tender and the mixture has thickened.
4. Turn off the heat and let it cool for a few minutes.
5. Divide the oatmeal into bowls, sprinkle nuts and fresh berries on top.
6. Go out and have fun!

_Greek Yogurt With Honey And Granola.

Ingredients
- 1 cup of Greek yogurt
- 2 tablespoons of honey
- 1/4 cup of granola.

Instructions
1. Put the Greek yogurt in a bowl. 2. Pour the honey over the yogurt and mix well.
3. Sprinkle the granola over the yogurt and honey mixture.
4. Serve and Enjoy!

_Scrambled Eggs With Spinach And Whole Grains Toast.

Ingredients
- 2 eggs
- 1/4 cup chopped fresh spinach
- Salt and pepper to taste
One slice of whole wheat bread

Instructions

1. Crack the eggs into the bowl and beat until well combined.
2. Heat a non-stick frying pan over medium heat.
3. Add the chopped spinach to the skillet and cook for 1-2 minutes, until tender.
4. Pour the beaten eggs into the pan with the spinach.
5. Use a whisk to stir the eggs until fully cooked.
6. Add salt and pepper to taste.
7. Toasted grain bread.
8. Put scrambled eggs on toast and enjoy!

_Smoothie Bowl With Mixed Berries And Chia Seeds.

Ingredients
1 cup mixed berries (fresh or frozen)
- 1/2 banana
- 1/2 cup of almond milk
- 1 teaspoon of chia seeds
- 1 teaspoon of honey (optional)

Toppings: sliced fresh fruit, granola, shredded coconut, extra chia seeds

Instructions
1. In a blender, combine the berries, banana, almond milk, chia seeds, and honey (if using).
2. Blend at high speed until smooth and creamy.
3. Pour the juice into a bowl.

4. Garnish with fresh fruit slices, granola, shredded coconut and add chia seeds if desired.
5. Serve and Enjoy

_Avocado Toast With Smoked Salmon.

Ingredients
- 1 avocado
- 1/4 lemon juice
- Salt and pepper to taste

Two slices of whole wheat bread
2 ounces smoked salmon
- 1 tablespoon of chopped fresh dill on top .

_Keep moving and have fun.

Instructions
1. Cut the avocado in half, remove the pot, and pour the pulp into a bowl.
2. Put the lemon juice, salt, and pepper in a bowl and mash with a fork until smooth.
3. Toast whole grain bread.
4. Spread the mashed butter over each slice of toast.
5. Place the smoked salmon on top of each slice of toast.
6. Sprinkle the chopped fresh dill on top.
7. Get moving and have fun!

_Quinoa Breakfast Bowl With Fruit And Nuts.

Ingredients
- 1/2 cup of quinoa

- Cup water
1/2 cup mixed berries (fresh or frozen)
1/4 cup chopped nuts (such as almonds, pecans, or walnuts)
Half a banana, cut into slices
- 1 teaspoon of honey (optional)

Instructions
1. Wash the quinoa well through a fine sieve.
2. Fill medium_sized pot, with water and bring to a boil over high heat .
3. Add the quinoa and reduce the heat .
4. Cover and simmer for 15-20 minutes or until water is absorbed and the quinoa is tender.
5. Crush the quinoa with a fork and divide it into two bowls.
6. Garnish each bowl with the berry mixture, chopped nuts, banana slices, and a little honey (if using).
7. Get moving and have fun!

_Whole Grain Waffles With Peanut Butter And Banana.
Ingredients
- 1 cup whole wheat flour
- 1 tablespoon baking powder
- 1/4 teaspoon of salt
- A cup of milk
- 1 egg
- 2 tablespoons of melted butter
- 1/2 cup creamy peanut butter

Banana cut into slices

Instructions

1. In a large mixing bowl, whisk together the whole wheat flour, baking powder, and salt.
2. In another bowl, whisk the milk, eggs and melted butter.
3. Pour the wet ingredients into the dry ingredients and stir to combine.
4. Preheat the waffle maker and coat with cooking spray.
5. Pour the batter into the waffle maker and bake according to the manufacturer's instructions.
6. Spread peanut butter on each cake and arrange banana slices on top.
7. Get moving and have fun!

_Breakfast Burrito With Scrambled Eggs And Black Beans.

Ingredients
- 4 large eggs
- 1/4 cup of milk
- Salt and pepper to taste
- 1 tablespoon of olive oil
- 1 can black beans, drained and rinsed
- 1/2 teaspoon dill
- 1/2 teaspoon of chili powder
- 4 large flour buns
- 1/2 cup grated cheddar cheese
- Sauce to serve

Instructions
1. In a mixing bowl, whisk together the eggs, milk, salt, and pepper.
2. Heat the olive oil in a large saucepan over medium heat.
3. Put the egg mixture in the pan and stir until cooked.
4. In another pan, heat the black beans with the cumin and chili powder until the beans are tender. 5. Reheat the tortilla in the microwave or in the skillet.
6. To wrap the burrito, place a spoonful of scrambled eggs and black beans on each tortilla.
7. Sprinkle the shredded cheddar cheese over the eggs and beans. 8. Roll up the tortilla, tucking in on the sides as you roll.
9. Serve with salsa, if desired. Enjoy!

_Cottage Cheese With Fruit And Honey.
Ingredients
- 1 cup of cheese
1/2 cup of fresh fruit mix (such as berries, sliced peaches, or chopped mango)
- 1 tablespoon of honey

Instructions.
1. In a mixing bowl, mix the cheese, fresh fruit, and honey.
2. Stir gently until everything comes together.
3. Eat as soon as possible or keep in the refrigerator until ready to serve. Enjoy!

Veggie Omelet With Whole Grain Toast.

Ingredients.
- 2 eggs
1/4 cup chopped vegetables (such as peppers, onions, mushrooms, or spinach)
- 1 tablespoon of olive oil
- Salt and pepper to taste
One slice of whole wheat bread

Instructions:
1. In a small bowl, beat the eggs with a fork.
2. Heat the olive oil in a non-stick frying pan over medium heat.
3. Add the chopped vegetables to the pan and sauté for 2-3 minutes, until tender.
4. Pour the beaten eggs over the vegetables in the skillet.
5. Using a spoon, gently lift the edges of the omelet and let the uncooked egg flow to the bottom. 6. When the omelet is almost done, fold it in half and place it on a plate.
7. Toast slices of whole grain bread.
8. Serve the omelet with toast on the side. Enjoy!

LUNCH.

1. Grilled Chicken Breast Topped With Quinoa And Mixed Vegetables.
2. Baked Salmon With Sweet Potato And Asparagus .
3. Lentil Soup With Carrots, Celery And Spinach.
4. Grilled Turkey Burger With Avocado And Tomato Salad.
5. Vegetable Stir-Fry With Tofu Brown Rice.
6. Baked Sweet Potato With Black Beans, Salsa And Greek Yogurt.
7. Grilled Portobello Mushroom Burger With Side Salad.
8. Minestrone soup with crackers
9. Grilled shrimp skewers with vegetables and grilled couscous
10. Chicken breast stuffed with spinach and feta cheese served with baked sweet potato.

_Grilled Chicken Breast Topped With Quinoa And Mixed Vegetables.

Ingredients.
1 boneless, skinless chicken breast
- 1/2 cup of quinoa
1 cup of mixed vegetables (carrots, broccoli, cauliflower, peppers)
- 1 teaspoon of olive oil
- 1/2 teaspoon garlic powder

- 1/2 teaspoon onion powder
- Salt and pepper to taste.

Instructions.

1. Rinse the quinoa and place it in a bowl with 1 cup of water. Once boiling, reduce heat and cover. Cook for 15 to 20 minutes or until water is absorbed and quinoa is tender.
2. Heat the griddle or baking sheet over medium-high heat.
3. Marinate the chicken breasts with garlic powder, onion powder, salt and pepper. Grease it with a little olive oil.
4. Bake the chicken for 6 to 7 minutes on each side or until just cooked through.
5. While the chicken is cooking, chop the mixed vegetables into small pieces.
6. Add olive oil to a frying pan and heat over medium heat. Add the mixed vegetables and sauté for 5-7 minutes or until tender.
7. To serve, place the cooked quinoa on a plate or bowl. Pour the vegetable mixture over the top, then the grilled chicken breast on top.
8. Serve immediately and garnish with fresh herbs, if desired.

This dish is rich in protein and fiber, which is very important for cancer patients. Quinoa is an excellent source of complex carbohydrates and contains all nine essential amino acids. Mixed greens provide a variety of vitamins and minerals, as well as antioxidants that help protect against cancer. Grilled chicken breast is a source of lean, easily digestible protein and contains important nutrients such as B vitamins and zinc.

Baked Salmon With Sweet Potatoes And Asparagus.

Ingredients:
- 1 salmon filet
- 1 large sweet potato
- 1 bundle of asparagus
- 1 lemon
- 1 tbsp olive oil
_Salt and pepper to taste.

Instructions
1. Preheat the oven to 200°C.
2. Wash the sweet potato and cut it into small cubes. Spread them out on a baking sheet and drizzle them with olive oil. Season with salt and pepper.
3. Bake the sweet potatoes in the oven for 15-20 minutes, or until tender.
4. While the sweet potato is baking, prepare the salmon. Place the salmon filet on a baking sheet and season with salt and pepper.
5. Cut the lemon in half and squeeze the juice over the salmon filet.
6. Bake the salmon in the oven for 15-20 minutes, or until cooked through.
7. Wash the asparagus and cut off the woody ends. Drizzle with olive oil and season with salt and pepper.

8. Add the asparagus to the baking sheet with the sweet potatoes and continue baking for 10-12 minutes, or until the asparagus is tender.
9. Once everything is cooked, serve the salmon filet with the sweet potato cubes and asparagus. Drizzle with lemon juice and enjoy!

Note: It is important to consult with a healthcare professional or a dietitian to determine the specific dietary needs and restrictions for a cancer patient.

_Lentil Soup With Carrots, Celery And Spinach.
Ingredients.
One piece of salmon filet
- 1 large sweet potato.
_A bunch of asparagus
- 1 lemon
- 1 tablespoon of olive oil
- Salt and pepper to taste.

Instructions
1. Preheat the oven to 200°C.
2. Wash the potatoes and cut them into small squares. Spread it on a baking sheet and drizzle it with olive oil. Season with salt and pepper.
3. Bake the sweet potatoes for 15-20 minutes or until tender.
4. While the sweet potatoes are cooking, prepare the salmon. Place the salmon filet on a baking sheet and season with salt and pepper.

5. Cut a lemon in half and squeeze the juice over the salmon filets.
6. Bake the salmon for 15 to 20 minutes, or until cooked through.
7. Wash the asparagus and cut off the stem. Drizzle with olive oil and season with salt and pepper.
8. Place the asparagus in the baking tray with the sweet potatoes and continue cooking for 10-12 minutes or until the asparagus is tender.
9. Once everything is cooked, serve the salmon filets with the sweet potatoes and asparagus. Drizzle it with lemon juice and enjoy!

Note: It is important to consult with a healthcare professional or dietitian to determine the specific nutritional needs and limitations of a cancer patient.

_Grilled Turkey Burger With Avocado And Tomato Salad.
Preparing a roasted turkey and avocado luncheon burger for cancer patients can be a healthy and delicious meal option. Here are the steps to prepare this dish:

Ingredients
- 1 pound ground turkey
- 1 avocado
- 1 small onion, finely chopped
- 2 minced garlic cloves
- 1 teaspoon of salt
- 1/2 teaspoon black pepper

- 1 tablespoon of olive oil
Whole grain burger
Lettuce leaves
Tomato slices

Instructions

Firstly, Wash your hands well before you start cooking.
2. Preheat the oven to medium-high heat.
3. In a mixing bowl, combine ground turkey, chopped onion, minced garlic, salt, and black pepper. Mix well so that all ingredients are evenly distributed. 4. Divide the mixture into 4 equal parts and shape each part into a pancake.
5. Brush both sides of each pancake with olive oil.
6. Place the patties on a preheated tray and bake for 5-6 minutes on each side or until cooked through. 7. While waiting for the pancakes to cook, cut the avocado in half, remove the pit, and scoop the pulp into a small bowl.
8. Mash the butter with a fork until smooth and creamy.
9. Bake the whole wheat burger on the griddle for a minute or two, until slightly crispy.
10. To assemble the burger, place a leaf of lettuce on the bottom half of each bun, then a piece of cooked turkey, sliced tomato, and some grated avocado.

11. Cover the top half of the bread and serve immediately.

The Grilled Turkey Avocado Burger is a nutritious and delicious meal packed with protein, healthy fats, and fiber. It is also easy to digest and gentle on the stomach, making it the perfect choice for a cancer patient's lunch. Enjoy !

_Vegetables Stir Fry With Tofu Brown Rice.

Stir-fried tofu with vegetables and brown rice is a healthy and delicious meal option for cancer patients. Here are the steps to prepare this dish:

Ingredients.
1 block of firm tofu, cut into small squares
2 cups mixed vegetables (such as bell peppers, broccoli, carrots, mushrooms), chopped
- 1 small onion, chopped
- 2 minced garlic cloves
- 1 tablespoon of olive oil
- Salt and pepper to taste
- 2 cups of cooked brown rice.

Instructions.

Firstly, Wash your hands well before you start cooking.
2. Heat the olive oil in a large skillet over medium-high heat.

3. Add chopped onion and minced garlic to the pan and sauté for 1-2 minutes until fragrant.
4. Add the chopped vegetables to the pan and sauté for 3-4 minutes until crispy.
5. Add the tofu cubes to the pan and continue to sauté for another 2-3 minutes, until the tofu is slightly brown.
6. Add salt and pepper to taste.
7. Serve the stir-fry over a bed of cooked brown rice.

This vegetable stir-fry with tofu and brown rice is a nutritious, long-lasting meal that's rich in fiber, vitamins, and minerals. It is also low in fat and calories, making it an ideal meal choice for cancer patients who need to maintain a healthy weight. Enjoy!

_Baked Sweet Potato With Black Beans, Salsa And Greek Yogurt.

Here are the steps to prepare this dish:
Ingredients
- 1 medium sweet potato
- 1/2 cup canned black beans, drained and rinsed
- 1/4 cup of sauce
- 1/4 cup of Greek yogurt

Instructions
1. Preheat the oven to 200oC.
2. Wash the potatoes well and poke them with a fork.

3. Place sweet potatoes in a baking tray and bake for 45-60 minutes or until tender when pierced with a fork.

4. While the sweet potatoes are baking, prepare the toppings. In a small bowl, mix black beans and salsa.

5. When the sweet potatoes are tender, remove them from the oven and let them cool for a few minutes.

6. Cut the potatoes in half lengthwise and use a fork to scrape the skin off.

7. Pour black bean mixture and salsa over 1/2 sweet potato.

8. Cover each potato half with a layer of Greek yogurt.

These baked sweet potatoes topped with black beans, salsa, and Greek yogurt are a delicious, nutrient-dense meal packed with fiber, protein, and vitamins. It is also low in fat and calories, making it an ideal meal choice for cancer patients who need to maintain a healthy weight.

_Grilled Portobello Mushroom Burger With Side Salad.

Here are the steps to prepare this dish:

Ingredients
2 large portobello mushrooms
- 2 whole wheat burgers
- 1/4 cup balsamic vinegar
- 1 tablespoon of olive oil
- Salt and pepper to taste

- 2 cups of mixed vegetables
1/2 cup cherry tomatoes, halved
-1/4 of a purple onion, thinly sliced
1/4 cup crumbled feta cheese
-2 tablespoons of balsamic vinegar

Instructions

1. Heat the griddle or baking sheet over medium-high heat.
2. Wash the portobello mushrooms and remove the stems.
3. In a small bowl, whisk together the balsamic vinegar and olive oil. Spread the mixture on both sides of the mushrooms and season with salt and pepper.
4. Place the mushrooms on the grill and cook for 4 to 5 minutes per side, or until tender and grill marks appear.
5. While the mushrooms are baking, prepare the side salad. In a large bowl, mix the mixed greens with the cherry tomatoes, red onion, and feta cheese.
6. Pour the balsamic vinegar over the salad and mix well.
7. Bake the burger on the grill for a few seconds.
8. Assemble the burger by placing the roasted portobello mushrooms on the bottom half of each bun.
9. Put a generous amount of salad on top of each mushroom.

10. Place the top half of the burger on each burger and serve immediately.

The Grilled Portobello Mushroom Burger with Salad is a healthy and delicious meal packed with antioxidants, fiber, and protein. It is also low in fat and calories, making it an ideal meal choice for cancer patients who need to maintain a healthy weight.

Enjoy!

_Grilled Shrimp Skewers With Roasted Vegetable And Couscous.

Here are the steps to prepare this dish:

Ingredients

1 pound large shrimp, peel and devein.
- 1 red pepper cut into cubes
- One yellow zucchini cut into slices
- 1 zucchini cut into slices
- 1 small purple onion, cut into pieces
- 2 tablespoons of olive oil
- Salt and pepper to taste
- 1 cup of couscous
1 1/4 cups chicken or vegetable broth
- 1 tablespoon of butter
- 2 tablespoons of freshly chopped parsley

Instructions

Firstly, Preheat the oven to 200oc.
2. Shrimp on skewers alternating with bell pepper, zucchini, zucchini and red onion.
3. Brush the skewers with olive oil and season with salt and pepper.

4. Place skewers on a baking sheet and bake in the oven for 10 to 12 minutes or until shrimp are pink and cooked through evenly.
5. While the skewers are grilling, we prepare the couscous. In a medium saucepan, bring broth and butter to a boil.
6. Add the couscous, stir well, cover the pot and remove from heat.
7. Let the couscous rest for 5 minutes, then mash it with a fork.
8. Add the chopped parsley to the couscous and stir well.
9. Serve grilled shrimp skewers with grilled vegetables and couscous on the side. This meal is full of essential nutrients for cancer patients. Shrimp is a good source of protein and omega-3 fatty acids, roasted vegetables provide antioxidants and fiber.
Couscous is a good source of complex carbohydrates that can help maintain energy levels throughout the day. Enjoy!

_Minestrone Soup With A Side Of Whole Grain Crackers.

Ingredients
- 2 tablespoons of olive oil
- 1 onion, chopped
- 2 minced garlic cloves

Two medium carrots, chopped
- 2 stalks of chopped celery
- 1 medium-sized grain, chopped

1 cup green beans, peeled and cut into bite-sized pieces
1 can (14.5 ounces) diced tomatoes, undrained
4 cups of low-sodium chicken or vegetable broth
- 1 teaspoon dried basil
- 1 teaspoon dried oregano
Salt 1/2 tsp
- 1/4 teaspoon black pepper
1 can (15 ounces) cannellini beans, drained and rinsed
1 cup small pasta, such as ditalini or elbow macaroni
- 1/4 cup grated Parmesan cheese
Whole grain crackers, to serve

Instructions

1. In a large skillet or Dutch oven, heat the olive oil over medium heat.
2. Add the onion and garlic and cook for 5 minutes, until softened. 3. Add the carrots and celery and cook for another 5 minutes.
4. Add the zucchini and green beans and cook for an additional 3 minutes.
5. Add the tomato cubes, broth, basil, oregano, salt and pepper. 6. Bring to a boil, then reduce heat and simmer for 20 minutes.
7. Add the cannellini beans and pasta and simmer for another 10-12 minutes or until the pasta is tender.

8. Add Parmesan cheese and stir. 9. Serve hot minestrone with whole-grain crackers on the side. This is a meal rich in fiber, vitamins and minerals and is very important for cancer patients. The vegetables in the soup provide antioxidants and anti-inflammatories that may help boost the immune system and fight cancer cells. Whole grain crackers are a good source of complex carbohydrates that can help maintain energy levels. Enjoy!

_Chicken Breast Stuffed With Spinach And Feta Cheese Served With Baked Sweet Potato.

Ingredients
4 boneless, skinless chicken breasts
- 1 cup of chopped fresh spinach
- 1/2 cup of feta cheese
- 2 minced garlic cloves
- 1 tablespoon of olive oil
- Salt and pepper to taste
4 medium sized sweet potatoes, peeled and cut into cubes
- 1 tablespoon of honey
- 1 tablespoon of olive oil
- 1/2 teaspoon smoked paprika
- 1/4 teaspoon garlic powder

Instructions
1. Preheat the oven to 375 oc.

2. In a small bowl, mix together the chopped spinach, the grated feta cheese, the minced garlic, and the olive oil.
3. Use a sharp knife to make a hole in each chicken breast.
4. Stuff the spinach and feta mixture in each chicken breast.
5. Season the chicken breasts with salt and pepper.
6. Place the stuffed chicken breasts in the baking tray and bake for 25-30 minutes or until the chicken is cooked through.
7. While the chicken is boiling, prepare the baked sweet potato.
8. In a large bowl, mix the potato cubes with the honey, olive oil, smoked paprika, and garlic powder.
9. Spread the sweet potatoes in a single layer on a baking sheet.
10. Bake the sweet potatoes in the preheated oven for 20-25 minutes or until tender and lightly browned.
11. Serve spinach and chicken breast stuffed with feta cheese with roasted sweet potatoes. This is a meal rich in proteins, vitamins and minerals that are essential for cancer patients. Chicken provides lean protein that can help maintain muscle mass. The spinach and feta filling adds flavor and nutrients like calcium and vitamin K. Sweet potatoes are a good source of complex carbohydrates that can help maintain energy levels. Enjoy!

DINNER.

Here are 10 good dinner options for cancer patients:

1. Grilled chicken with grilled vegetables
2. Grilled salmon with quinoa and steamed broccoli
3. Lentil soup with salad
4. Spicy turkey with brown rice
5. Vegetable stir-fry with tofu brown rice
6. Roasted sweet potato, roasted chicken and green beans
7. Grilled Cod with Asparagus and Sweet Potatoes
8. Chicken curry with vegetables and brown rice
9. Grilled shrimp with grilled vegetables and quinoa
10. Grilled chicken with roasted brussels sprouts and sweet potatoes.

1_Grilled Salmon With Grilled Vegetables.

Grilled salmon with grilled vegetables is a tasty and healthy lunch option for cancer patients. Salmon is an excellent source of protein and omega-3 fatty acids, which are important for maintaining a healthy immune system. Roasted vegetables, such as broccoli and sweet potatoes, are full of vitamins and minerals that may help support overall health during cancer treatment.

Here's how to prepare this dish:

Ingredients
One piece of salmon filet
- 1/2 cup cherry tomatoes
- 1/2 cup of chopped broccoli
- 1/2 cup chopped sweet potato
- 1 tablespoon of olive oil
- Salt and pepper to taste

Instructions
1. Firstly, Preheat the oven to 200oC.
2. Put parchment paper on the baking tray.
3. Place the salmon fillet on the baking tray and season with salt and pepper.
4. In another bowl, mix cherry tomatoes, broccoli, and sweet potatoes with olive oil, salt, and pepper.
5. Arrange the vegetables around the salmon on a baking sheet.
6. Bake for 15 to 20 minutes or until salmon is cooked through and vegetables are tender.
7. Remove from the oven and let it cool for a few minutes before serving.

This meal can be served with brown rice or quinoa for more fiber and nutrients. It is important to consult with a healthcare practitioner or registered dietitian to ensure that this meal meets the patient's individual nutritional needs and limitations.

2_Lentil Soup With Salad.

Lentil soup with whole wheat bread is a comforting and nutritious dinner option for cancer patients. Lentils are an excellent source of protein and fiber, while whole grain bread provides complex carbohydrates that can help maintain energy levels during cancer treatment. Here's how to prepare this dish:

Ingredients
- 1 cup dried lentils
- 1 chopped onion
- 2 minced garlic cloves
- 2 chopped carrots
- 2 stalks of chopped celery
6 cups of vegetable broth
- 1 teaspoon of dill
- 1 teaspoon of chili powder
- Salt and pepper to taste
Whole grain bread, to serve

Instructions
1. Rinse the lentils in a colander and set aside.
2. In a large saucepan, sauté the onion and garlic in a little olive oil until soft.
3. Add the chopped carrots and celery to the pan and cook for a few minutes until they soften slightly.
4. Add the lentils to the pan and stir to combine with the vegetables.
5. Pour in the vegetable broth and add the cumin and paprika.

6. Bring the soup to a boil, then reduce heat and simmer for 30 minutes or until the lentils are tender.
7. Season with salt and pepper to taste.
8. Serve hot with whole wheat bread. This meal can be customized by adding other vegetables such as spinach or kale, or by using chicken or beef broth instead of vegetable broth. It is important to consult with a healthcare practitioner or registered dietitian to ensure that this meal meets the patient's individual nutritional needs and limitations.

3_Grilled Salmon With Quinoa And Steamed Broccoli.

Ingredients
4 boneless, skinless chicken breasts
- 1 cup of quinoa
Two cups of water
- 1 head of broccoli
- Salt and pepper to taste

Instructions for using olive oil:
1. Preheat the oven to 375 oc.
2. Wash the quinoa and put it in a saucepan with 2 cups of water. Bring to a boil, then reduce heat and simmer for 15 minutes.
3. While the quinoa is cooking, chop the broccoli and chop it into bite-sized pieces. Place the broccoli in a steamer and steam for 5-7 minutes, until tender.

4. Season the chicken breasts with salt and pepper. Heat a small amount of olive oil in a saucepan over medium-high heat. Fry the chicken breasts for 2-3 minutes on each side, until golden brown.

5. Transfer the chicken breasts to a baking dish and bake for 20-25 minutes, until cooked through.

6.Serve grilled chicken with cooked quinoa and steamed broccoli.

This meal is rich in protein and contains all the essential nutrients needed by cancer patients undergoing treatment. Quinoa is a good source of fiber that helps maintain a healthy digestive system.

Broccoli provides a variety of vitamins and minerals, including vitamin C and folic acid, that support the immune system. Chicken is a good source of lean protein, which helps repair and rebuild tissues damaged by cancer treatment.

4_Spicy Turkey With Brown Rice.

Ingredients
- 1 cup brown rice
Two cups of water
- 1 tablespoon of olive oil
- 1 onion cut into slices
- 2 minced garlic cloves
- 1 red capsicum, sliced
- 1 yellow capsicum, sliced
- 1 zucchini cut into slices
- 1 cup of broccoli
- 1 cup sliced mushrooms
1 tablespoon of low-sodium soy sauce
- 1 tablespoon of honey
- 1 teaspoon grated fresh ginger
- Salt and pepper to taste.

Instructions
1. Wash the brown rice through a fine sieve and place it in a medium saucepan with 2 cups of water. Bring to a boil, then reduce heat to low and cover the pan. Cook for 40 to 45 minutes or until the rice is tender and has absorbed the water.
2. While the rice is cooking, heat the olive oil in a large saucepan over medium-high heat. Add the onion and garlic and sauté for 2-3 minutes, or until the onion is translucent.
3. Add the peppers, zucchini, broccoli and mushrooms to the skillet and sauté for 5 to 7 minutes or until tender .

5_Vegetables Stir_Fry With Tofu With Brown Rice.

Ingredients:
- 1 block of firm tofu, drained and cubed
- 1 red bell pepper, sliced
- 1 yellow onion, sliced
- 2 cups broccoli florets
- 1 cup snow peas
- 2 cloves garlic, minced
- 1 tablespoon grated ginger
- 1 tablespoon olive oil
- Salt and pepper, to tasteFor the brown rice:
- 1 cup brown rice
- 2 cups water
- Salt, to taste

Instructions:
1. Rinse the brown rice in cold water and drain. In a medium saucepan, add the rice, water, and salt. Bring to a boil, then reduce the heat to low and cover the pot with a tight-fitting lid. Cook for 40-45 minutes, or until the rice is tender and the water is absorbed.

2. Heat the olive oil in a large pan over medium heat. Add the cubed tofu and cook for 5-7 minutes, or until browned on all sides. Remove the tofu from the skillet and set aside.

3. In the same pan, add the sliced bell pepper, sliced onion, broccoli florets, and snow peas.

Cook for 5-7 minutes, or until the vegetables are tender but still crisp.

4. Add the minced garlic and grated ginger to the skillet and cook for 1-2 minutes, or until fragrant.

5. Add the cooked tofu back to the skillet with the vegetables and stir to combine. Season with salt and pepper, to taste.

6. Serve the stir fry over the brown rice and enjoy!

Note: This recipe can easily be adapted to include other vegetables or protein sources based on the patient's preferences and nutritional needs. Be sure to consult with a healthcare professional or registered dietitian for personalized dietary recommendations.

6_Roasted Sweet Potato, Roasted Chicken And Green Beans

For a cancer patient, a dinner of roasted sweet potato, roasted chicken, and green beans can be a healthy and nutritious option.

It is important to ensure that the chicken is cooked thoroughly and that the sweet potato and green beans are seasoned with herbs and spices instead of sait.

1 Preheat the oven to 200°C.

2. Prepare the ingredients:
Wash and peel 2 medium sweet potatoes, then cut them into 1-inch cubes.
3.Rinse 4 boneless, skinless chicken breasts and pat dry with paper towels.
4.Wash and chop 450g of fresh green beans.
5.Sweet Potato and Chicken Seasoning:
In a large bowl, mix sweet potato balls with 1 tablespoon olive oil,
1 teaspoon dried rosemary leaves, 1 teaspoon dried thyme, and
1/4 teaspoon black pepper.

1.In another bowl, season the chicken breasts with 1 tablespoon of the olive oil,
2.1 tablespoon of the dried basil,
3.1 tablespoon of the dried oregano leaves, and
1/4 teaspoon of the black pepper.
4. Arrange the sweet potatoes and chicken on a large baking sheet, making sure they are evenly spaced and not overlapping.
5. Place the baking tray in the preheated oven and bake for 20 minutes.
6. While the sweet potatoes and chicken are baking, prepare the hummus:
In a bowl, mix the chickpeas with 1 tablespoon of olive oil,
1/2 teaspoon of garlic powder, and 1/4 teaspoon of black pepper.
7. After 20 minutes, remove the baking sheet from the oven, add the seasoned chickpeas,

and spread them evenly around the chicken and sweet potatoes.

8. Return the baking sheet to the oven and continue to bake for another 15 to 20 minutes or until the chicken reaches an internal temperature of 165°F (74°C) and the sweet potatoes are tender.

9. Remove the baking tray from the oven and let the food rest for 5 minutes.

10. Arrange the baked sweet potatoes, chicken, and green beans on a plate and serve immediately. Enjoy your nutritious and delicious meal!

7_Grilled Cod With Asparagus And Sweet Potatoes.

This recipe for Grilled Cod with Asparagus and Sweet Potatoes is a good option for cancer patients:

Ingredients
1 pound cod filet, skin on top
1 tablespoon of olive oil
1 teaspoon of salt
1/2 teaspoon black pepper
1 bunch of asparagus, trimmed
1 sweet potato, peeled and diced
1/4 cup of lemon juice
1 tablespoon chopped fresh dill

Instructions

1.Heat the grill over medium heat.
In a small bowl, mix the olive oil, salt, and pepper.
2.Rub the mixture over all of the cod filets.
3.Place the asparagus and sweet potatoes on a baking sheet and drizzle the lemon juice over the top.
4.Bake the cod filets for 4 to 5 minutes on each side or until just cooked through.
5.Bake the asparagus and sweet potatoes for 10 to 12 minutes, or until tender.
6.To serve, place the cod filet on a serving platter and garnish with the asparagus and sweet potatoes.
7.Sprinkle with dill. This dish is a good source of protein, vitamins and minerals, and is low in fat and calories. Cod is a good source of omega-3 fatty acids, which have been shown to have anti-cancer properties. Both asparagus and sweet potatoes are good sources of fiber, which can help keep your digestive system healthy.
Here are some tips when preparing this dish for cancer patients:

Use fresh fish with a mild flavor. Cook the fish until done.
Served with fish and simple, easy-to-digest vegetables. Avoid using strong spices or sauces.

8_Chicken Curry With Vegetables And Brown Rice.

Here is a recipe for chicken curry with vegetables and brown rice that is perfect for a cancer patient:

Ingredients:
1 tablespoon olive oil
1 onion, chopped
2 cloves garlic, minced
1 inch piece of ginger, peeled and minced
1 teaspoon turmeric powder
1 teaspoon coriander powder
1 teaspoon cumin powder
1/2 teaspoon garam masala
1/2 teaspoon cayenne pepper
1 pound boneless, skinless chicken breasts, cut into 1-inch pieces
1 (14.5 ounce) can diced tomatoes, undrained
1 (15 ounce) can chickpeas, rinsed and drained
1 (10 ounce) package frozen peas
1 cup brown rice, cooked

Instructions:
1. Heat the olive oil in a large skillet over medium heat.
2. Add the onion, garlic, and ginger and cook until softened, about 5 minutes.
3. Add turmeric, coriander, cumin, garam masala and chilies and cook for another minute.
4. Add the chicken and cook until golden on all sides.

5. Add diced tomatoes, beans and peas. Bring to a boil and cook for 15 minutes or until chicken is completely cooked through. 6. Served on brown rice.

This recipe is a good source of protein, fiber, and complex carbohydrates, all of which are important for cancer patients. Turmeric, ginger and other spices found in curry also have anti-inflammatory properties, which may benefit cancer patients.

To make this recipe more crab-friendly, you can use low-sodium canned tomatoes and chickpeas, and you can omit the chilies if you prefer a milder curry. You can also serve the curry with yogurt or sauce.

Enjoy!

_Grilled Shrimp With Grilled Vegetable And Quinoa.

Ingredients

1 medium shrimp, peeled and deveined
- 1 large zucchini, cut into slices
- 1 large red bell pepper, sliced
- 1 large yellow bell pepper, sliced
- 1 large purple onion, chopped
- 2 tablespoons of olive oil
- 1 teaspoon of salt
- 1 teaspoon black pepper
- 1 teaspoon garlic powder
- 1 cup of quinoa
- 2 cups of water

Instructions
1. Preheat the oven to medium heat.
2. In a large bowl, mix the shrimp, zucchini, chilies, and shallots with the olive oil, salt, black pepper, and garlic powder.
3. Thread shrimp on skewers and set aside.
4. Place the vegetables on the grill and cook for 10-15 minutes or until soft and slightly charred, stirring occasionally.
5. Grill the shrimp for 2-3 minutes on each side, until the shrimp are cooked through and turn pink.
6. Meanwhile, rinse the quinoa under cool running water. In a medium saucepan, bring water to a boil over high heat. Add the quinoa and reduce the heat to low. Cover and simmer for 15 to 20 minutes or until the water is completely absorbed.
7. Serve grilled shrimp and vegetables on a bed of quinoa.

This meal includes cancer-fighting ingredients such as turmeric in a smoothie (not in dinner) and nutrient-dense vegetables in the main course. It's also high in shrimp and quinoa proteins, which can aid in muscle recovery during treatment.

_Grilled Chicken With Roasted Brussels Sprouts And Sweet Potatoes.

Roasted Chicken with Brussels Sprouts and Roasted Sweet Potatoes Recipe:

Ingredients

For the grilled chicken:
- 2 boneless chicken breasts
- 1 tablespoon of olive oil
- 1 teaspoon garlic powder
- 1 teaspoon of chili powder
Salt 1/2 tsp
- 1/4 teaspoon black pepper

For the Brussels Sprouts and Baked Sweet Potato:

2 cups Brussels sprouts, trimmed and cut in half
2 cups sweet potatoes, peeled and cut into small cubes
- 2 tablespoons of olive oil
- 1 teaspoon garlic powder
- 1 teaspoon dried thyme
Salt 1/2 tsp
- 1/4 teaspoon black pepper

Instructions

1. Preheat the oven to 200C.
2. In a small bowl, mix the olive oil, garlic powder, paprika, salt, and black pepper. Brush the chicken breasts with the mixture on both sides.

3.Heat a grill pan over medium heat and grill the chicken for 6-7 minutes on each side or until cooked through.

4.While the chicken is cooking, prepare the roast vegetables. In a large bowl, mix the Brussels sprouts, sweet potatoes, olive oil, garlic powder, thyme, salt, and black pepper until the vegetables are evenly coated.

5.Spread the vegetables in a single layer on a baking tray and bake in the oven for 20-25 minutes or until tender and lightly browned.

6.Serve the grilled chicken with roasted Brussels sprouts and sweet potatoes.

This recipe is rich in fiber, protein and vitamins, which makes it a healthy and nutritious meal option for everyone, especially cancer patients.

SMOOTHIE.

Green Smoothie.
Mango and Ginger Smoothie.
Avocado Smoothie.
Turmeric Smoothie.
Blueberry Smoothie.
Chocolate Smoothie.
Blueberry and Almond Smoothie.
Beetroot Smoothie.
Ginger Smoothie
Berry Smoothie

1 Green Smoothie.

It's great when you're looking to help a cancer patient through nutrition. Green juice can be a great way to get the nutrients your body needs. Here is a healthy green smoothie recipe suitable for cancer patients:

Ingredients:
1 cup baby spinach
1/2 cup shredded kale
1/2 cup frozen mango
1/2 cup unsweetened almond milk 1 tablespoon ground flaxseed
1/2 teaspoon grated fresh ginger Instructions

Place spinach and kale in a blender and blend until finely chopped.
Add mangoes, bananas, almond milk, flaxseeds, and ginger root in a blender.
Pour in a glass and enjoy!

2. Mango And Ginger Smoothie.

Ingredients
- 1 ripe mango, peeled and chopped
- A small piece of fresh ginger, peeled and chopped
1 cup of unsweetened almond milk
- 1 tablespoon of honey
- 1 cup of ice cubes

Instructions
1. Place the mangoes and ginger in a blender.
2. Pour in the almond milk and honey.
3. Add ice cubes.
4. Blend at high speed until the juice is completely smooth.
5. Taste and adjust sweetness as needed by adding honey.
6. Pour into a glass and enjoy!

3. Avocado Smoothie.

However, here is a simple avocado smoothie recipe that can be modified to meet the nutritional needs of cancer patients:

Ingredients
A ripe avocado
- 1 banana

1 cup almond milk (or other milk substitute)
1 tablespoon honey (or any other sweetener)
- 1/2 teaspoon of vanilla extract
Optional: ice cubes

Instructions
1. Cut the avocado in half and remove the seeds. Remove the meat and put it in the blender.
2. Peel the banana and put it in the blender.
3. Add the almond milk, honey, and vanilla extract to the blender.
4. If you like, you can add ice cubes to the blender for an even cooler smoothie.
5. Mix all ingredients until smooth and creamy.
6. Pour the juice into a glass and enjoy it right away.

Note: Depending on the nutritional needs of the cancer patient, you may need to modify this recipe by removing some ingredients or replacing them with others. It is best to consult a dietitian or healthcare professional before making any significant changes to a cancer patient's diet.

4. Tumeric Smoothie.

Ingredients
1 cup of unsweetened almond milk
A frozen banana
- 1/2 teaspoon turmeric powder
- 1/2 teaspoon ground cinnamon
- 1/2 teaspoon of ginger powder
- 1 tablespoon of honey
- 1/4 teaspoon black pepper

Ice cubes (optional)

Instructions.
1. Put the almond milk, frozen banana, turmeric powder, cinnamon powder, ginger powder, honey, and black pepper into a blender.
2. Blend until smooth and creamy. 3. If desired, add ice cubes and blend again until smooth.
4. Pour into a glass and enjoy your turmeric drink !

5.Blueberry Smoothie.

Ingredients

- 1 cup of frozen blueberries
Small banana
1/2 cup plain Greek yogurt
- 1/2 cup of almond milk
- 1 tablespoon of honey
- 1 teaspoon of chia seeds

Instructions
1.Wash all parts thoroughly before use.
2. Place the blueberries, bananas, Greek yogurt, almond milk, honey, and chia seeds in a blender.
3.Mix the ingredients until smooth.
4. Pour the juice into a glass and serve immediately.
Blueberry juice is rich in antioxidants and anti-inflammatory compounds that may help reduce cancer risk and support the immune

system. It is also a good source of protein, fiber, and healthy fats that can provide energy and nutrition for cancer patients undergoing treatment.

6. Chocolate Smoothie.

Ingredients
- 1 ripe banana
1 cup of unsweetened almond milk
- 1 tablespoon of cocoa powder
- 1 tablespoon of honey
- 1/2 teaspoon of vanilla extract
- 1/2 cup of ice

Instructions
1. Peel the banana and cut it into pieces.
2. Place the banana pieces, almond milk, cocoa powder, honey and vanilla extract in a blender.
3. Mix the ingredients until smooth.
4. Add ice to the blender and blend again until the smoothie reaches the desired consistency.
5. Pour the juice into a cup and use it right away.

Instructions
- Use ripe bananas to make sweet smoothies.
-Adjust the amount of honey according to your taste.
 -If the juice is too thick, add more almond milk or water. -
You can add other ingredients like chia seeds, flaxseeds, or protein powder to make the smoothie more nutritious.

7. Blueberry And Almond Smoothie.

However, here is a simple blueberry and almond drink recipe that can be modified to meet the nutritional needs of cancer patients:

Ingredients

- 1 cup of frozen blueberries
- 1 banana
1 cup of almond milk (or any other milk substitute)
1 tablespoon of honey (or any other sweetener)
- 1/2 teaspoon of vanilla extract
Optional: ice cubes

Instructions

1. Put the frozen blueberries into a blender.
2. Peel the banana and put it in a blender.
3. Put the almond milk, honey and vanilla in a blender.
4. If desired, add some ice cubes to the blender for an even cooler smoothie.
5. Mix all ingredients together until smooth and creamy.
6. Pour the juice into a glass and enjoy it right away.

Note: Depending on the nutritional needs of the cancer patient, you may need to modify this recipe by removing some ingredients or substituting them with alternative ingredients. It is best to consult a dietitian or healthcare professional before making any significant changes to a cancer patient's diet.

8. Beetroot Smoothie.

Ingredients
- 1 radish of medium size, peeled and chopped
- 1 small, peeled and chopped islands
- 1 small, square and chopped apple
1 cup of fresh spinach leaves
Fresh ginger 1/2 inch, peeled and grind
1 teaspoon of honey
1 cup of water or almond milk

Instructions
1. Wash all the ingredients carefully before using them.
2. Place the beets, carrots, apple, spinach leaves, grated ginger and honey in a blender.
3. Pour in water or almond milk.
4. Mix the ingredients until smooth.
5. Pour the juice into a cup and use it right away.
Beetroot juice is full of antioxidants, vitamins, and minerals that can help boost the immune system and fight cancer cells. It is also a great source of fiber, which can aid in digestion and promote overall health.

9. Ginger Smoothie.

Ingredients
1 inch of fresh ginger root
- 1 banana
A cup of frozen pineapple

1 cup of unsweetened almond milk
- 1 tablespoon of honey
- Half a teaspoon of vanilla extract
- 1 cup of ice cubes

1. Peel and grate the ginger root. 2. Place the ginger, banana, frozen pineapple, almond milk, honey and vanilla extract in a blender.
3. Mix all ingredients together until smooth.
4. Add ice cubes and blend again until smooth.
5. Pour the ginger juice into a glass and enjoy!

Optional: Add a scoop of protein powder for an extra protein

Berry Smoothie.

Ingredients:
- 1 cup frozen mixed berries
- 1/2 banana
- 1 cup unsweetened almond milk
- 1 tablespoon honey
- 1 teaspoon vanilla extract

Instructions:

1. In a blender, combine the frozen mixed berries, banana, almond milk, honey, and vanilla extract.

2. Blend until smooth.

3. Pour the smoothie into a glass and serve.

7 MEAL PLAN DAYS.

Day 1:
Breakfast: oatmeal with bananas in slices, almond milk and chia seeds
- Snack: apple slices with almond butter
Lunch: quinoa salad with grilled vegetables, green beans and feta cheese
- Snack: carrots stick to the net
Dinner: grilled salmon with grilled potatoes and green beans

Day 2.
Breakfast: Greek yogurt with mixed berries and granola.
- Snack: Mix the tracks with nuts and dried fruits.
Lunch: Turk and a lawyer with wheat tortilla.
- Snack: cheese with slices
Dinner: breaking vegetables with brown rice and tofu.

Day 3:
Breakfast: Eggs are sad of spinach and toys whole wheat
Snack: Edamame Bean
Lunch: lens soup with beans biscuits completely
Snack: Greek yogurt with honey and nuts
Dinner: chicken oven with grilled cauliflower and quinoa

Day 4.
Breakfast: fruit juice with frozen fruit, bananas, Greek milk, almond milk and chia seeds
- Snack: rice cakes with peanut butter and banana
Lunch: Spinach salad with grilled chicken, strawberry and fun
- Snack: cut into Tzatziki sauce
Dinner: the secret of pasta with Turkey and Marinara sauce

Day 5:
Breakfast: Gall of whole grains with fresh fruits and plants
- Snack: green beans bread
Lunch: grilled cheese sandwich with tomato soup
-Snack: apple slices with cinnamon
_Dinner: a slice cooked with grilled asparagus and sweet potatoes

Day 6:
Breakfast:
Toast for lawyers with solid eggs and cherry tomatoes
- Snack: Hummus with Pita Closet Simice
Lunch:Tuna salad with mixed green vegetables and wheat biscuits
- Snack: Greek yogurt with mixed berries and granola

_Dinner: Grilled salmon with grilled Brussels and wild rice

Day 7:
Breakfast:
Fruit juice with frozen fruit, Greek milk and granola
- Snack: Mix the tracks with nuts and dried fruits
Lunch: Ceasar Chicken Salad with whole grain bread
-Snack: pepper slices with a guaranteed farm
_Dinner: Luza mixed vegetables with additional salad.

SNACKS FOR CANCER PATIENTS.

Some ideas for healthy and nutrient-dense snacks for cancer patients:

1. Apple slices with almond butter
2. Greek yogurt with berries and honey
3. Hummus with carrots and cucumber slices
4. Trail mix with nuts, seeds and dried fruits
5. Boiled eggs with biscuits
6. Cheese slices with peach or pineapple
7. Edamame (soybeans) with sea salt
8. Avocado toast on whole wheat bread
9. Marinated Roasted Green Beans
10. Homemade granola bar with oats, nuts and dried fruits.

OTHER SIMPLE RECIPES FOR CANCER PATIENTS.

Here are some simple recipes that may be included in a cancer cookbook for beginners:

1. Creamy Broccoli Soup

Ingredients:
- 2 cups broccoli florets
- 1 onion, chopped
- 2 cloves garlic, minced
- 4 cups low-sodium chicken broth
- 1 cup heavy cream
- Salt and pepper, to taste

Instructions:
1. In a large pot, sauté the onion and garlic until softened.

2. Add the broccoli and chicken broth to the pot and bring to a boil.

3. Reduce heat and simmer until the broccoli is tender.

4. Use a blender or immersion blender to puree the soup until smooth.

5. Add the heavy cream and stir to combine.

6. Season with salt and pepper to taste.

2. Grilled Chicken Salad

Ingredients:

- 2 boneless, skinless chicken breasts
- 6 cups mixed greens
- 1 cup cherry tomatoes, halved
- 1 avocado, sliced
- 1/4 cup crumbled feta cheese
- 2 tablespoons olive oil
- 2 tablespoons balsamic vinegar
- Salt and pepper, to taste

Instructions:

1. Preheat a grill or grill pan to medium-high heat.

2. Season the chicken breasts with salt and pepper.

3. Grill the chicken for 5-6 minutes per side, or until cooked through.

4. Let the chicken rest for a few minutes before slicing into bite-sized pieces.

5. In a large bowl, combine the mixed greens, cherry tomatoes, avocado, and feta cheese.

6. In a small bowl, whisk together the olive oil, balsamic vinegar, salt, and pepper.

7. Pour the dressing over the salad and toss to combine.

8. Divide the salad onto plates and top with the sliced chicken.

3. Berry Smoothie

Ingredients:

- 1 cup frozen mixed berries
- 1/2 banana
- 1 cup unsweetened almond milk
- 1 tablespoon honey
- 1 teaspoon vanilla extract

Instructions:

1. In a blender, combine the frozen mixed berries, banana, almond milk, honey, and vanilla extract.

2. Blend until smooth.

3. Pour the smoothie into a glass and serve.

CHAPTER SEVEN.
CONCLUSION.

A cancer diagnosis can be overwhelming, but there are many ways to take control of one's health during treatment. A cancer cookbook for beginners can provide patients with healthy, delicious recipes that support their bodies during treatment. These recipes can help patients manage side effects, maintain their strength and energy levels, and feel more in control of their health. With the help of a cancer cookbook, patients can enjoy flavorful meals that nourish their bodies and support their overall well-being.

Printed in Great Britain
by Amazon